Surviving Chronic Pancreatitis

What Every Veteran Needs to Know

Joseph Henry Morsette MSCJA, JD, LL.M.

Indigenous Combat Two-Service U.S. Veteran

USAF Staff Sergeant; USA Private First Class

Is-pi-mik-ki-ew High Eagle

PUBLISHED BY: Joseph Henry Morsette, High Eagle Coaching and Consulting Services, LLC.

DISCLAIMER AND/OR LEGAL NOTICES

While all attempts have been made to verify information provided in this book and its ancillary materials, neither the author or publisher assumes any responsibility for errors, inaccuracies, or omissions and is not responsible for any financial loss by customer in any manner. Any slights of people or organizations are unintentional. If advice concerning legal, financial, accounting, or related matters is needed, the services of a qualified professional should be sought. This book and its associated ancillary materials, including verbal and written training, is not intended for use as a source of legal, financial, or accounting advice. You should be aware of the various laws governing business transactions or other business practices in your particular geographical location.

EARNINGS & INCOME DISCLAIMER

With respect to the reliability, accuracy, timeliness, usefulness, adequacy, completeness, and/or suitability of information provided in this book, Joseph Henry Morsette, Joseph Henry Morsette, High Eagle Coaching and Consulting Services, LLC, its partners, associates, affiliates, consultants, and/or presenters make no warranties, guarantees, representations, or claims of any kind. Readers' results will vary depending on a number of factors. Any and all claims or representations as to include earnings are not to be considered as average earnings. Testimonials are not representative. This book and all products and services are for educational and informational purposes only. Use caution and see the advice of qualified professionals. Check with your accountant, attorney, or professional advisor before acting on this or any information. You agree that Joseph Henry Morsette and/or Joseph Henry Morsette, High Eagle Coaching and Consulting Services, LLC, is not responsible for the success or failure of your personal, business, health, or financial decisions relating

Printed in THE UNITED STATES OF AMERICA

Cover Design by Tashai Lovington

MOTIVATE AND INSPIRE OTHERS!

"Share This Book"

Eight Reasons why you should buy this Book in Bulk:

1. **REWARD** those who have helped your group by giving them a FREE autographed book;
2. **INVEST** in your community, your inner circle;
3. **INCREASE ATTENDANCE** by advertising that the first "X" number of people attending your event receive a FREE autographed book;
4. **DOOR PRIZES**: Give the books away as door prizes;
5. **BOOK SIGNING**: Advertise that Joseph will be autographing books after the event to increase attendance;
6. **RAISE MONEY FOR YOUR GROUP** by selling the books at your event for the full retail price;
7. **INCREASE EVENT VALUE** by incorporating the cost of the book for every participant into your registration fee; and
8. **AUTOGRAPH SESSION**: Joseph will conduct a special autograph session to sign all of the books at no cost,

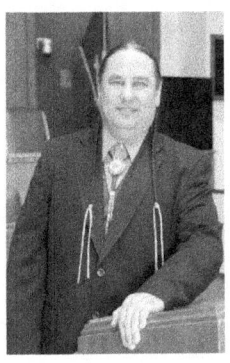

Retail $14.95

Special Quantity Discounts
NO Taxes, and NO Shipping & Handling

5-50 Paperback Books - $13.00
51-99 Paperback Books - $11.00
100-499 Paperback Books - $10.00
500-999 Paperback Books - $9.00
1,000+ Paperback Books - $8.00

To Place an Order Contact Joseph:
www.HighEagleLLC.com

THE IDEAL PROFESSIONAL
SPEAKER FOR YOUR NEXT EVENT!

Any organization that wants to develop their people to become "extraordinary," needs to hire Joseph for keynote and/or workshop training!

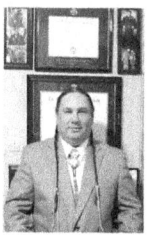

TO CONTACT OR BOOK JOSEPH TO SPEAK:
Joseph Henry Morsette,
High Eagle Coaching and Consulting Services, LLC
www.HighEagleLLC.com

THE IDEAL CONSULTANT FOR YOU!

If you are ready to overcome challenges, have major breakthroughs, and achieve higher levels, then you will love having Joseph as your consultant!

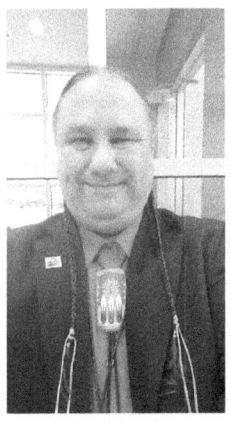

TO CONTACT OR BOOK JOSEPH TO CONSULT:
Joseph Henry Morsette,
High Eagle Coaching and Consulting Services, LLC

www.HighEagleLLC.com

Dedication

It is with great respect, admiration, and sincere appreciation, that I dedicate this book to my wonderful family. To my great-grandparents, my grandparents, my parents, my wife, my children, and my grandchildren.

To my wife, Juanita Benally Morsette for driving me to the hospital on many occasions, and saving my life. Without you, I would not be here today, to share the blessings of family. I love you dearly.

Contents

Foreword

My name is Major Ed Pulido, U.S. Army (Ret.). I am the Founder of the John-Daly Major Ed Heart of a Lion Foundation with PGA Professional Mr. John Daly. Additionally, I am the former Sr. VP, Co-Founding member of Folds of Honor Foundation and Co-Founder of Warriors for Freedom Foundation. Finally, I am the Author of "Warrior for Freedom: Challenge, Triumph, and Change." An autobiography by Major Edward Pulido, as told by Marie Bartlett.

My story begins on August 17th, 2004, when I was hit by an Improvised Explosive Devise (IED) or roadside bomb in Baquobah, Iraq that would change my life forever. As I laid on the 128-degree heat, one thing was clear, as a member of the Armed Forces of the United States of America, we all understand that it is our patriotic duty to never leave a fallen comrade behind on the field of battle and on the Homefront, so help us God.

It was at that moment in the heat of battle, that I would remember what my Hispanic immigrant father and Vietnam War combat Veteran Chief Warrant Officer

Manuel Pulido once told me. He told me that when you take the oath of office to defend the greatest nation in the world, it is about God, Country, Family, and all of those that serve in the Armed Forces of the United States America to protect you, the American people.

For years, the United States of America has always honored the military men and women who have sacrificed so much for our freedoms. It is this devotion and sacrifice that has truly been the bedrock of our sovereignty as nations, our values as people, our security as democracies, and our offer of hope to those in other lands who dream of freedom, of "Life, Liberty, and the Pursuit of Happiness."

It is in that spirit of service and sacrifice, that I first met Joseph at the Oklahoma VetWorks 2022 Annual Conference, where I was the Keynote Speaker. Joseph is a great man and an outstanding patriot! His can-do-attitude to help others struggling, and tenacity to lift up his fellow man is above reproach. That was the main reason that I decided to write this Foreword, and support Joseph with this inspiring book.

If you wanted to know what the signs are of necrotizing chronic pancreatitis, how to get immediate care, and how to follow-up with your primary care, then this book is for you and your family. It's what I call the mission first and people always approach to giving back and paying it forward to those living with this debilitating disorder. A progressive inflammatory disorder that leads to irreversible destruction of exocrine, and endocrine pancreatic parenchyma caused by atrophy, and/or replacement with fibrotic tissue.

In this book you will read about the challenges, triumphs, and changes in Joseph's journey. Just like my autobiography, in this book you will experience the spirit of love, hope, and faithful purpose. As I see it, there is something compelling when someone has gone through a life-threatening event such as I did when I hit that roadside bomb. One thing is clear, you learn quickly who is on your side and more importantly you learn that it is in God's hands from this day forward.

It is in that spirit, that I want to share with you these powerful verses that inspired me on my journey, but inspire Joseph in his walk-in life to give back to those that need love, hope, and wisdom.

Greater love hath no man than this, that a man lay down his life for his friends."

John 15:13

"Even though I walk through the valley of the shadow of death, I will fear no evil, for you are with me; your rod, and your staff, they comfort me."

Psalm 24:3

"For God so loved the world, that he gave his only Son, that whoever believes in him should not perish but have eternal life."

John 3:16

"Blessed is the one who perseveres under trial because, having stood the test, that person will receive the crown of life that the Lord has promised to those who love him."

James 1:12

Major Edward Pulido, U.S. Army, (Ret.)
CEO, John Daly-Major Ed Heart of a Lion Foundation
OEF and OIF Combat Veteran
Purple Heart Recipient

A Message To You!

I was lying in bed at the VA hospital when the phone rang. It was my father. He told me that CNN was broadcasting a story about an Army Veteran who had just died from pancreatitis, a treatable disease, because he could not get an ICU bed.

The news hit hard, not just because of the tragedy itself, but because of the systemic failure it represented. It wasn't just a single veteran lost; it was a symptom of a larger issue affecting many. The realization that this could have been me, or one of my friends, brought a wave of determination crashing over me. I felt overwhelmed by a sense of urgency and responsibility. That was when the idea of telling my story came to me.

A couple of days later, I saw the same news story on the TV in my hospital room. From my bed, I opened my phone and took this photo.

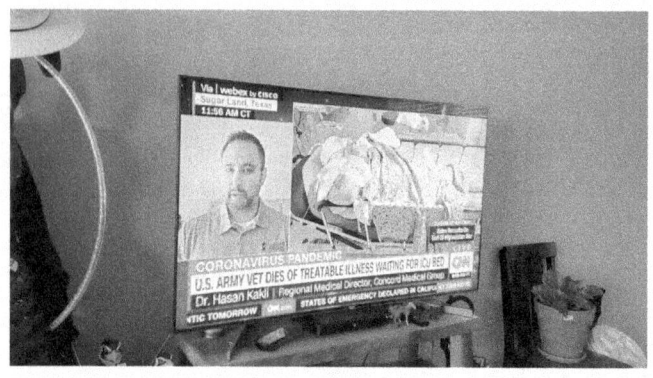

It was right then that I decided it was my mission to write this book, retelling my story of surviving chronic pancreatitis. Then the rest of the book needed to be about helping other U.S. Veterans to recognize the signs of chronic pancreatitis, how to get access to an emergency room, and finally how to follow through at home with the recommendations from their medical team.

The days that followed were filled with reflection and planning. I documented every detail of my medical journey, the early symptoms I had ignored, the misdiagnoses, the frustrations, and the eventual breakthrough. I recalled the times I felt isolated and scared, not knowing where to turn for reliable information or support. These memories were painful, but they fueled my resolve.

As I lay there in the sterile, cold environment of the hospital, the news of the Army Veteran's death haunted me. The ceiling tiles became a checkerboard of thoughts and memories, each square filled with fragments of my journey. The IV drip's rhythmic beeping was a constant reminder of my own vulnerability, tethering me to the reality of my illness and the precariousness of life.

I imagined the book as a lifeline, a beacon of hope and

knowledge for veterans grappling with similar health issues. It would be more than just my story; it would be a comprehensive guide, a step-by-step manual for navigating the complexities of the medical system. I envisioned chapters dedicated to recognizing early symptoms, understanding the importance of timely medical intervention, and navigating the often-confusing bureaucracy of VA hospitals.

In my quiet moments, I jotted down ideas and outlines, kept track of the timeline of events. Each word was a promise to my fellow veterans: I will help you. I will share my knowledge, my experiences, and my strength. Together, we can overcome this.

With every passing day, my determination grew stronger. This book would be my legacy, a testament to resilience and the power of shared knowledge. It would be a call to action, urging veterans to take charge of their health and seek the help they deserve.

God blesses you to bless others. I set out to write this book as a survival guide with you in mind—the United States Veteran—and to serve you. On December 12, 2020, and again seven months later on June 29, 2021, I came within one hour of dying. But for the Grace of God, through my wife, my Earth-Angel Juanita Benally Morsette, I survived chronic necrotizing pancreatitis (CNP). As a survivor of this horrific ordeal, I want to empower you with my strategies, techniques, and outcomes to go from where you are to where you want to be. I hope to inspire you into new ways of thinking differently about thriving with whatever form of pancreatitis you may be experiencing.

Sharing my story has been good therapy. I pushed myself to get out of bed and stay up longer and longer every day as I researched and wrote this book. It has helped me fill in some, but not all, the days and weeks that have gone by over the past three years since my first gallstone attack in January 2020.

My story includes my inner circle of support, my team, my village. They are made up of my family, close friends, colleagues, and medical doctors, nurses, and other staff who have helped me get through a very tough but manageable road to my recovery. Their support has given me the right mindset to continue, it's not over. I am able to take it one day at a time rather than fighting for my life second by second, minute by minute, hour by hour.

I am here to share with you:

- my story,
- the signs for recognizing pancreatitis,
- how to access VA and non-VA health care,
- how to follow up with your primary care medical team of doctors, nurses, and other staff,
- how having CNP changed my life.

What does this mean for you? I want to thank you personally for your service to our country, our beautiful and wonderful nation. I stand at attention and salute you. It does not matter where you are in life; I want to help you gain a better understanding of being learned in what is chronic pancreatitis. Every fellow Veteran deserves to have the necessary and proper care when facing a treatable medical condition. Nobody gets left behind. We are all in this together.

It is my hope that this story not only inspires you but also reminds you that you are not alone. You do not have to battle this illness by yourself. As you power through this new chapter in your life, there is a medical team, a village, waiting to assist you if you let them.

I offer life-changing takeaways after each chapter. This book is my gift to you.

Giga Waabamin Miinawaa Chi-Migwetch (Thank you very much; we will see each other again), from the Anishinaabe language.

Chapter 1
EVERYTHING IS SPINNING

From what I can now remember, the following is a timeline of my firsthand experience dealing with the symptoms of CNP. Although I had trouble recalling details at the time, later I obtained much of the information from my daily journals, speaking with my immediate family, and referring to my medical records.

Prior to 2020, I thought I was doing fine. My mindset and my health were okay. I felt good. I was eating anything that I wanted to eat. I exercised daily. I am not an alcohol user. I am not a drug user. I traveled back and forth to my job as an in-house legal counsel for the legislative branch of the Cheyenne Arapaho Tribes. I worked a full-time schedule of forty hours a week. I was able to do daily chores for myself and others. There were no signs of diabetes in my immediate family, including my father, my mother, and siblings. Later, I would learn that people with pancreatitis have a greater risk of developing type 2 diabetes, and the opposite is true as well.

I thought, overall, my health was fine. Sure, I was a little overweight for my height and age but nothing to be too concerned about. I saw my primary care doctor once a year as is recommended. I had a prescription for heartburn, high blood pressure, and some as-needed pain medication. Both Juanita and I felt the dosage for the first two was more than I needed, and so we wanted to talk to my physician about having the prescription reduced. Still, I considered myself to be in good health.

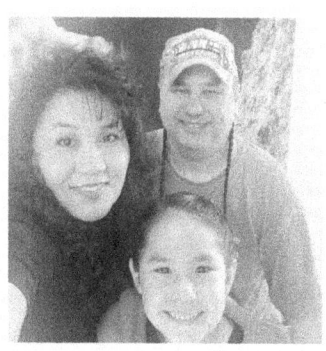

It all began in January of 2020. I was bloated and experiencing severe pain in my stomach and on the right side of my abdomen. I remember that first time driving myself to the emergency room at the Oklahoma City Veterans Affairs Medical Center (OKC VAMC). I was on the interstate, and things were getting a little scary. It was a 20 minute ride, and as I'm driving, I'm getting lightheaded. I'm feeling dizzy, nauseated, and like I was going to vomit. I'm thinking, "Where can I pull over?" It's five or six lanes by the time you get into the city, and to be feeling this way was legitimately alarming. I started to panic a little, but then a space opened up and I was able to get to the side of the road. I immediately threw up. It was such a relief just to be able to pull over. But as I sat there, still bent over dry heaving while cars whizzed by, I was feeling like, "What's going on with me? This is really terrible!" Little did I know that this same thing was going to hit me over and over for the next three months.

At OKC VAMC, I passed my first gallstone. This would happen again and again. Severe pain and vomiting, another trip to the hospital, more gallstones. And after staying only a few hours each visit, they would send me home. During this three month period, no medical staff ever said, "Let's get your gallbladder removed."

Due to the COVID-19 pandemic, by mid March 2020, the OKC VAMC was only performing surgeries for severe conditions such as heart bypasses. They were not seeing routine walk-in patients. This could be the reason they did not make a recommendation for the removal of my gallbladder. And I never bothered to follow up with my primary care physician to ask whether or not gallbladder surgery was an option for me. The OKC VAMC did not contact me either. So as a result, they did not suggest any further medical care such as an x-ray, an exam on my stomach, or surgery to have my gallbladder removed. A lot of what happened to me after this could have been avoided if there would have been additional communication between me and my primary care physician.

This is why I strongly recommend that you take charge in regards to your own well-being. You need to follow up with your local VA medical team, whether they contact you first or not. Please be proactive with your health care!

I will never forget being jolted awake from my sleep. It was around 2:00 a.m. and the room was spinning. I called to my wife, Juanita, who was in our daughter's room that night.

I told her, "Everything is spinning!" My life was about to be turned upside down!

The date was December 12, 2020, almost a year removed from that first gallstone episode, but this was a hundred times worse. I was now hurting so bad that my abdomen felt like it was on fire! It was so bloated that I looked seven months pregnant. Again I was throwing up, and the pain was so bad that I was delusional. I don't even remember what all I said to my wife that night when she, along with my little daughter, Justice, drove me to the emergency room. It was some crazy trip. We had to stop along the side of the road again for me to vomit. I told Juanita that I didn't think I could hold on long enough for the full 20 minute drive from home to the VA hospital. So she instead took me to the nearest emergency room which turned out to be the Integris Canadian Valley Regional Hospital in Yukon, Oklahoma.

She dropped me off at the entrance to the hospital and went to park the car. I could barely walk by this time and practically crawled up to the intake desk. I was on my knees because I could no longer stand. There was a young girl at the counter, her first day on the job. She was having a hard time trying to input my information. I had to repeat it to her three times. Then Juanita came in from parking the car and finished giving her my details. I immediately moved as quickly as I could for the bathroom to vomit again. I was then admitted into the emergency room.

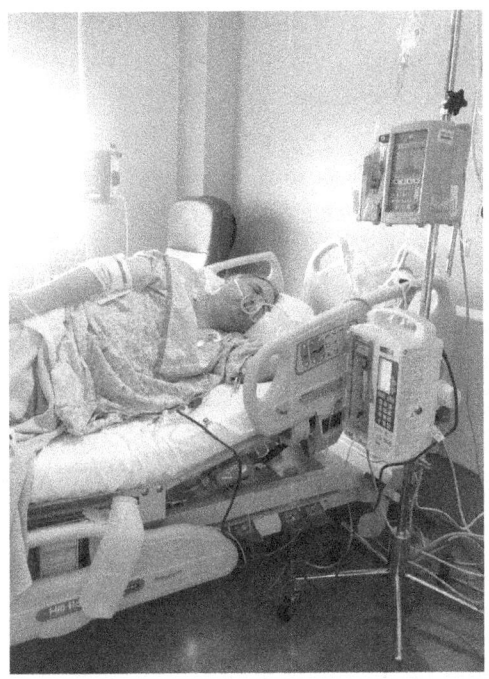

Two days later I was transported to Integris Baptist Medical Center in Oklahoma City where they would keep me for testing and observation over the next two weeks. My check-in weight was 240 pounds. They gave me morphine for the pain and conducted a series of tests. I don't remember what all they were because I was seriously out of it. I do remember them attempting an MRI, but the first machine they had me in ended up being too small. My belly was so bloated that I wouldn't fit. They had to transfer me to a larger one.

After all the tests, I still didn't know what was wrong with me. No mention of pancreatitis was made, but rather, they just thought I was passing more gallstones. I wanted to stay longer until I reached full recovery, but on Christmas

Day, the on-call doctor said that I was to be released. The hospital discharged me and sent me home. I was given medication to last a short period of time, but I do not remember specifically what my diagnosis was besides *passing gallstones*. And unfortunately, I was not yet in any condition to be proactive towards following up with the medical team to learn more.

Just a week or two later in early January 2021, Juanita and Justice once again drove me to the emergency room at OKC VAMC. And again, I do not remember much of what transpired. I blacked out on the way to the hospital. I do recall coming to while I was on an emergency room bed. One of the nurses told me to drink a lot of orange juice. Apparently, my blood sugar had dropped dangerously low.

The VA hospital called in a whole team of specialists and that's when they finally determined that I had chronic pancreatitis, However, the team of doctors could not operate. They informed me that my gallbladder was shooting gallstones at my pancreas like a pinball machine. There was too much damage for the surgeons to go in right away. I would need to wait until my body produced mature saturated bubbles around my pancreas before the damaged tissues could safely be removed. Otherwise, if they were to attempt surgery now, it would rupture my stomach. They were able to line things up with a specialist at the University of Oklahoma Medical Center (OUMC) who would perform these delicate procedures on me when my body was ready.

On January 15, 2021, I was discharged from the OKC VAMC and sent home with medication. I now weighed in at 194 pounds; that's a loss of 46 pounds in just 33 days.

Between January 30 to March 27, I would be admitted to either the OUMC or the OKC VAMC on numerous and separate occasions where I underwent procedures that consisted of putting me under anesthesia and scraping out the dead pancreas cells from my body. I would then spend several days at a time in the hospital recovering from each procedure. I was sent home after my recovery days, mostly to rest, and I was usually given an approximate two-week follow-up date to come back for another procedure. All in all, I believe it took seven procedures (and possibly more, I lost count) to finally get the dead pancreas cells removed from my body.

When I was first admitted to OUMC in January, I weighed 185 pounds. As the months rolled on, I continued the in and out at the OUMC and OKC VAMC hospitals. But now I required a feeding tube to be inserted into my stomach because the doctors did not want me eating anything on my own. From the end of March through August, my weight kept fluctuating. At my lowest point on April 25, I weighed in at just 138 pounds. That's a loss of 102 pounds in approximately 120 days.

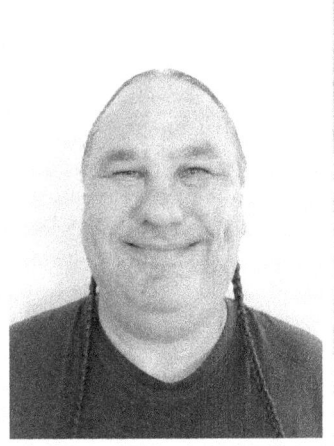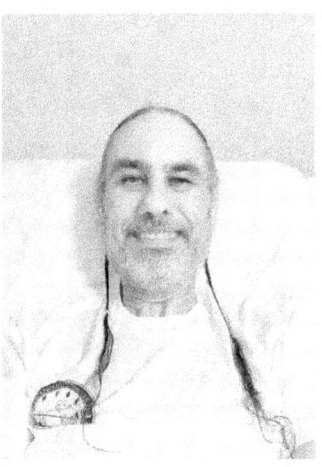

During this time, I was amazed at how I was actually still able to work. It was January 2020 and as a result of the pandemic, we went all-online. With no need to appear in person anymore, I could still perform all my work duties as legal counsel. Luckily, with the shut down, there were no court cases. All I had to do was text virtual meetings via phone and Zoom calls for three days per week.

My family, my sister, and my wife all assisted me with my recovery in so many ways, including driving me to all of my appointments. I was so weak after every hospital visit, I couldn't walk or really do anything for myself. Although I had a wheelchair, my condition was so severe that for the majority of the time, all I could do was lay in bed. Not even strong enough to get up to go to the bathroom, I was resigned to wearing diapers and using a bottle to urinate in. Talking was another issue. Unable to speak clearly, I found myself stuttering and slurring my speech. I would repeat things but not really say exactly what I wanted to get across.

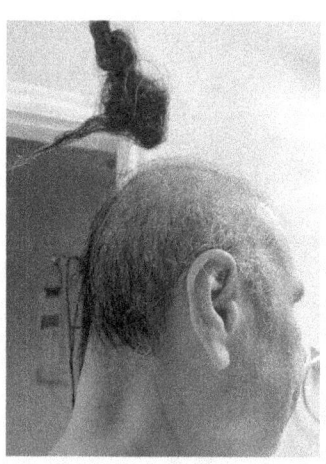

I ended up loosing all my hair. And it wasn't long before

I hit my rock bottom. As I said, Juanita and my family were helping me tirelessly, but they could only do so much and weren't able to be with me at all times. The reality of my situation was that I was alone for a good part of each day. I'm not too proud to say that I started having suicidal thoughts. Doubts would creep in, "What is all this for? Am I even getting any better?" I just wasn't sure it was worth it anymore. The truth is, I was so weak, even negative thoughts like these were just too much for me to sustain, which in hindsight is a good thing. Everything was an effort.

It's at times like these that you need to find your *why*. Why are you here? What is your reason for continuing the fight? Whether it's for you or someone else, having a purpose to live here and now on this planet can make all the difference. Lying in bed, hour by hour, day by day, I had to make a conscious decision to want to live. And it wasn't hard for me to find *my* why. My wife, young daughter, my grown children, and my other family members–they were my reason to live.

The turning point came when I started to see that my condition might actually have a chance to improve. It was only a little at first but then slowly I could do more. Walking was still incredibly hard to attempt. I had to lift my leg up with my hands from underneath just to get it to move, but at least I could do it. The OUMC provided me with a fancy walker with a seat, and then OKC VAMC issued a cane. These physical aids, along with a belief on my part, helped me to learn to walk again at home. Eventually, I made enough progress that I could abandon the wheelchair while going to my doctor appointments.

Call to Action!

Don't know your reason for living? These questions may help.

1. Name one goal that you want to accomplish today.
2. What are three goals that you want to achieve in the coming six months?
3. Write out one goal that you'd like to reach by this time next year?
4. Where do you want to be in your life in five years?
5. If you could achieve anything, but it would take ten years to reach it, what would it be?

Chapter 1 - Takeaways:

1. Remember the importance of taking charge of your own well-being. Your health is precious and being proactive in managing it can make a world of difference. Paying attention to your body and seeking medical attention when needed can be life-saving.

2. Don't hesitate to reach out to your healthcare providers and follow up on any concerns or symptoms you may have, even if they don't initiate the communication. Your actions could lead to early detection and prevention of serious complications.

3. Find your *why* and make a conscious decision to want to live. Life can throw you into dark moments, but your *why* can be a guiding light. Whether it's your family, friends, or your own personal aspirations, having a purpose to live can give you the strength to face any challenges that come your way.

Chapter 2
THE ROAD TO RECOVERY

My only desire was to be able to get up and move around, but my whole body was extremely sore. I had to learn how to do the most basic of things all over again, simple body functions that I had taken for granted my entire life. For instance, before I was to be discharged, I had to accomplish a series of tasks that, at the time, proved quite difficult for me. Things that should have been simple, such as coughing, farting, peeing, pooping (this was especially hard for me since I was not eating anything), and walking. This last task was also very challenging because the medical team always had me hooked up to at least two IVs and several machines that monitored my heart, lungs, and blood pressure.

There were so many different tests performed on me that I cannot remember when the doctors finally figured out what was actually going on with my body, nor what the specific test or symptom was that clued them in. My memory from this time period is a bit spotty, although I do recall one particular odd event that occurred. A nurse from the VA came into my room, wheeled me out in a wheelchair, and started down the hallway. We got as far as the front desk on that floor when we were met by the day doctor. She asked the nurse where she was taking me because no procedures or tests had been ordered for me that day. The nurse checked her notes, and it was determined that she had the wrong patient. Yikes! I was quickly returned to my room where I was supposed to be having a rest day.

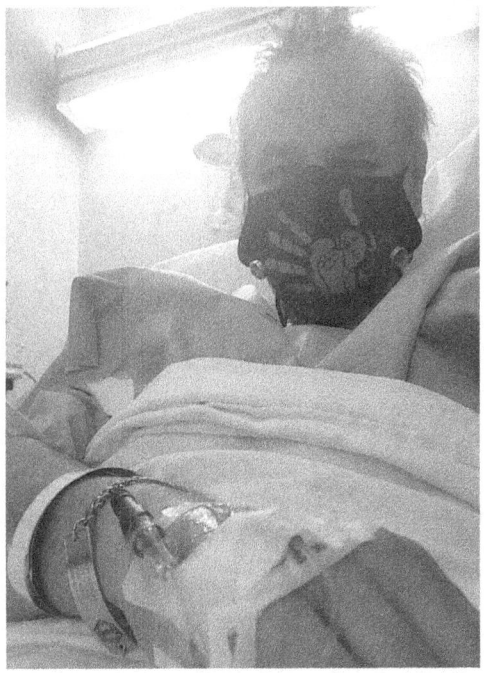

I would recommend that you always politely ask the nurses and doctors if you are the right patient that they are seeking and what type of procedure or test they will be performing on you that day. Again, it's important that you be proactive in your own healing journey. Don't be afraid to speak up and ask questions.

In April of 2021, the OKC VAMC contracted with Encompass Home Health Care to provide a nurse to come to my house to assist me with physical therapy twice a week. In addition, another nurse was there once a week for medical care. This service would continue for the next eight months until mid December.

On August 19, I was able to meet my weight goal of 160 pounds. Juanita and I returned for an office visit with my primary care specialist doctor at the OUMC. This is the surgeon who performed the seven-plus procedures on me. Today, he was going to remove my feeding tube so that I could now attempt to transition to eating solid foods. He was happy to see the progress I'd made, especially because, he told me, that on two separate occasions during those earlier procedures, I came within one hour of dying. He also said that if only I had come to him sooner, he might have been able to save my pancreas. This made me sad, but I was happy to be alive.

By the end of August, my body weight continued to show promise as I weighed in at 164 pounds. The doctors and nurses told me that because my gallbladder had destroyed my pancreas, my body was no longer able to produce insulin naturally. As a result, I would now have to take synthetic insulin moving forward. For the first time in my life, I was prescribed Glargine, a long-acting insulin, and Novolog Aspart, the short-acting version. I immediately did not accept this as the only answer. God has the final say. If he wants to repair my pancreas, then He will. In the meantime, I asked all of my doctors if a pancreas transplant was a possibility. One said that yes, it is possible, although it is usually done with a kidney transplant. My kidneys are really healthy, so there was no use trying to go that route. I will just have to wait for an artificial pancreas transplant or continue to take insulin for the remainder of my natural life. No matter what materializes, I am alive and happy to be here.

My medical team did an A1C analysis on me. It is a test that measures your average blood sugar levels over the course of three months. In addition to A1C, it can be referred to as hemoglobin A1C, glycated hemoglobin, or HbA1c. It is used to diagnose prediabetes or diabetes. If you already have diabetes, it monitors how you have been managing your blood sugars over a long period of time. The higher the A1C number, the higher your blood sugars have been running. Low A1C numbers mean a low blood sugar count. My A1C at this time was 12.2 which is high. I needed to be down to 7.0 or lower.

It was at the end of September that I was notified by the OUMC that I had tested positive for COVID-19. Up to that point, I had been checked 21 times, and all results came back negative. I'd received three Pfizer vaccinations prior to this. Now I had the virus, but gratefully, I didn't show any symptoms. My wife, daughter, and father-in-law all tested negative. My weight continued to improve and was now up to 177 pounds.

I was finally on the mend. By October 26, my A1C was down to 10.0. I weighed 181 pounds. On December 6, the A1C had dropped to 8.1 and my body weight was up to 191. A week later, I enrolled in a program at the OKC VAMC. It was an arthritis seated group exercise which I attended in person three times a week. Then out of convenience for me and less travel time, I enrolled in the online program which allowed me to participate from home. My weight was up to 195 pounds. By late December, I was enrolled in a once-a-week program for physical and occupational therapy at the Yukon VA Clinic in Yukon, Oklahoma.

With the coming of 2022, it was clear that I would not be able to return in person as an in-house legal counsel for the Cheyenne Arapaho Tribes. I simply could no longer engage in a substantial gainful activity eight hours a day, five days a week. The new speaker of the Legislature relieved me of my consulting duties, and I began to draw unemployment. As a result, I lost my civilian health care coverage with Blue Cross Blue Shield. My weight increased to 199 pounds.

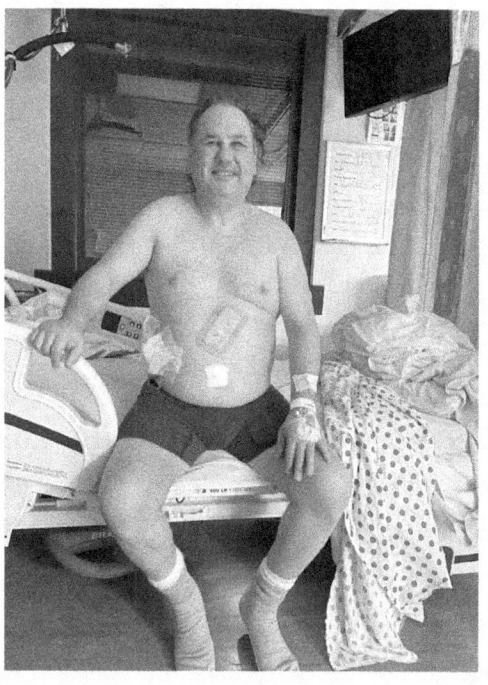

In March, I was admitted to the OKC VAMC for two

separate procedures, to have my gallbladder removed and my feeding tube hole repaired. The surgeries were a success, and I would be discharged two days later. When they weighed me, however, I was now up to 212 pounds. Not my ideal weight of 170.

I was tiring of having my weight go up and down, the rebound weight gain, and the yo-yo diets. In April, I hit 219 on the scale. So I started researching bariatric surgery which involves surgical adjustments to the digestive system to aid in weight loss. Because I am on high blood pressure medication, having this procedure would help to aid in controlling my blood sugar. I might even be able to reduce the amount of insulin I take. And it would definitely give me more confidence, help change my behavior on food portioning, and increase my energy towards improving my health for life. I watched a video at the OKC VAMC on the details of bariatric surgery. In it they discussed two different procedures: 1) a lower risk operation called sleeve gastrectomy where part of the stomach is removed and the remaining portion is fashioned into a long thin tube; and 2) another reliable, yet higher risk operation is referred to as the gastric bypass. The stomach is altered to hold less food with less weight-gain being the result. This is the method I am pursuing. As a requirement, I enrolled into VA MOVE which is a weight management and health promotion program for Veterans.

It was at this time that my primary care doctor wrote a detailed letter with my official medical diagnoses. It was as follows:

- pancreatic insufficiency
- pancreatic necrosis
- diabetic peripheral neuropathy

- type 2 diabetes
- kidney stones
- cholecystitis
- sleep apnea
- decreased muscle strength
- functional gait abnormality
- nutritional disorder
- atrial fibrillation
- oropharyngeal dysphagia
- coronary artery disease
- left knee patella chondroplasty
- gastroesophageal reflux disease
- vitamin D deficiency
- osteoarthritis
- disorder of refraction and/or accommodation
- orchialgia
- foot pain
- pes planus
- spermatocele
- repair of inguinal hernia
- tinnitus
- chronic post-traumatic stress disorder
- hypertension

For the rest of 2022, they continued to monitor my blood sugar and body weight. In mid July, my A1C was 7.4. I weighed 212 pounds. In August I successfully graduated from the VA MOVE program. I no longer needed a walker and was slowly weaning myself from the reliance on a cane. I can now walk on my own. My weight was 210. In September, my A1C was up a little to 7.8 as was my weight at 216 pounds. In October I was officially going through the

OKC VAMC checklist for bariatric surgery. Weight back down to 212.

And finally on October 19, I started receiving a combined service-connected rating of 100% from the VA. I am now considered to be totally and permanently disabled solely due to my service-connected disabilities. These disabilities include many of the conditions from my medical diagnosis above as well as bilateral hearing loss, post-traumatic stress disorder (PTSD) with depression and anxiety, chronic fatigue syndrome, and migraine headaches. The VA back-dated their decision from December 18, 2021. NOTE: I was honorably discharged from the military in 2004, but it was not until 2011 that I first applied for a VA service-connected disability rating. It only took me eleven years to go from 0 to 100%.

Separately, the Social Security Administration would find that I became disabled under their rules in June 2023, though they would only backdate my benefits to April.

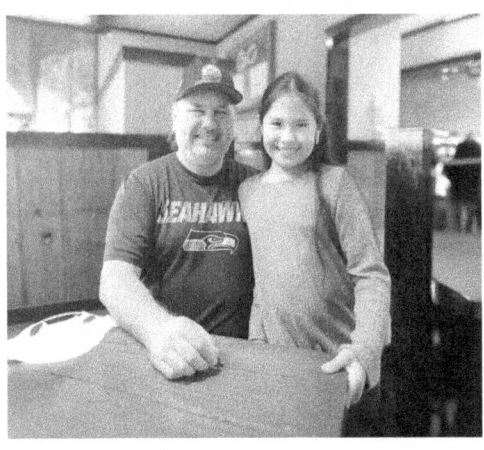

As I write this, it is now August 2023. My healing

journey has been long and one I could not have completed without both my dedicated medical team and my loving family. But I now have my life back, and I don't take a minute of it for granted. Remember to be proactive with your own healing journey. Talk to your doctors, follow up after checkups, and find *your* reason for living.

Chapter 2 - Takeaways:

1. When you are facing health challenges, it's very common to feel overwhelmed and isolated. Healthcare providers are dedicated to helping you through difficult times. Reaching out to them for assistance is a vital step towards recovery.

2. Take charge in regards to your own well-being. This involves actively engaging with your healthcare providers, asking questions, and seeking clarity on medical conditions, treatments, and procedures. Being informed empowers you to make better decisions about your health and ensures that you fully understand your treatment plans.

3. It may take some time, but if you stick with it, you can remake your life.

Chapter 3
WHAT IS CHRONIC PANCREATITIS?

I believe that everything in life has been done for me, not against me, and likewise for you, not against you. If you are currently experiencing chronic pancreatitis, I once walked in your shoes. I am a living testament that this illness, this disease, does not have to define you. It does not define me, nor does it confine me.

Maybe you are going through it, experiencing a pretty rough ordeal over a short span of time. Metaphorically, for every stone (kidney stone or gallbladder stone), there is a blessing. I believe illness cannot ever live, nor thrive in the living body of Christ. Have faith my friend. You are not alone.

When this happened to me, I had no idea what pancreatitis was. So let's go back to basic training.

What is a pancreas?

The pancreas is an organ that sits behind your stomach. It is an elongated gland, about one-and-a-half inches wide and approximately six to ten inches in length. It runs horizontally across the upper abdomen, but because it's hidden deep within the body, any medical diagnostics must be done with the use of imaging tech, e.g., CT scan, MRI, ultrasound, endoscopy.

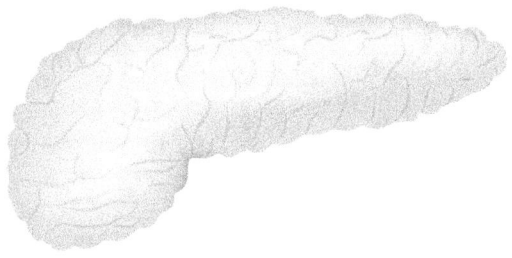

What does the pancreas do?

The pancreas has two main functions within the body. First, it produces digestive enzymes which are released into the small intestine. When you digest food, these enzymes are what breaks down carbs, fats, and proteins. In addition, the pancreas also produces hormones such as insulin and glucagon. These two guys work in harmony to regulate your blood sugar level, keeping it from drifting too high or too low.

What is pancreatitis?

Pancreatitis refers to a condition when the pancreas becomes inflamed and swollen. This swelling affects the gland's ability to release the digestive enzymes into the intestine. Instead, these enzymes get stuck inside the pancreas where they start to digest the very organ that created them.

The swelling causes the pancreatic ducts to squeeze

shut. As the enzymes build up, they simply do what they were designed to do—digest. They begin to munch away on the pancreas itself, a process called autodigestion.

Just think about how painful that can be. The pancreas, meant to aid in digestion, is now turning on itself. And as this inflammation keeps going, acinar cells keep doing what they do—churning out and activating the digestive enzymes, which in turn can then leak around the islet cells (which produce hormones). If this occurs, things may get even worse. Insulin and other hormones can be released directly into the bloodstream.

When these activated enzymes enter the blood, they can spread throughout the body, causing trouble wherever they settle. It's a real struggle for anyone who might be dealing with this condition.

What is chronic pancreatitis?

Chronic pancreatitis is ongoing inflammation of the pancreas. When this happens, the swelling typically does not heal and usually worsens over time. This condition also typically leads to damage and scarring of the pancreas.

Chronic pancreatitis commonly arises following one or multiple acute pancreatitis episodes. However, it can be triggered by just a single acute attack that leads to damage in the pancreas and its ducts.

With the buildup of scar tissue, the pancreas is slowly destroyed over time. As the pancreas is being attacked, bouts of pain typically come and go in people afflicted with this condition.

What are the symptoms of pancreatitis?

Abdominal pain is the primary and most frequent symptom of pancreatitis. Typically, this pain manifests as a sharp, stabbing sensation in the upper center of the abdomen. It tends to worsen after eating, especially with fatty foods or any type of beverage, including water.

Along with the pain, swelling and tenderness may develop in the abdomen. Activities like walking or lying down can also intensify the pain, while leaning or bending forward often provides some relief. Many individuals also experience sharp back pain which can be constant and severely debilitating.

Other symptoms of pancreatitis may include but are not limited to:

- bloating in the stomach
- swollen belly
- nausea and vomiting
- abdominal tenderness
- low blood pressure
- glucose intolerance
- bleeding from the pancreas causing a bluish discoloration of the abdomen
- jaundice-yellow eyes/skin
- weight loss due to poor digestion
- muscle spasms in arms and legs
- low calcium level
- chills
- clammy or sweaty skin
- rapid heart rate
- dehydration
- sweating

- chronic diarrhea
- tiredness
- fever
- dyspepsia
- weakness
- fatty or oily stools
- dizziness
- gaps in memory or memory loss
- amnesia
- chronic fatigue

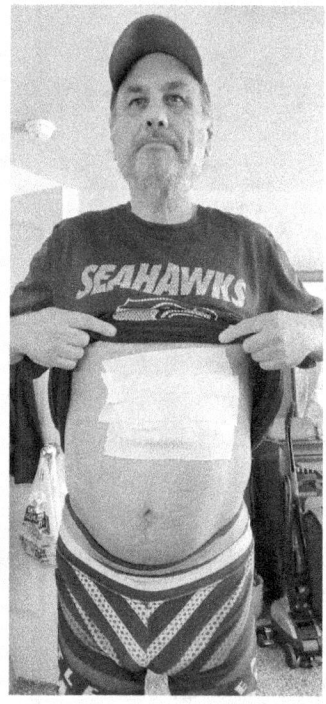

What are the causes of pancreatitis?

The most common cause of chronic pancreatitis is alcoholism, and for acute pancreatitis, it is gallstones. These small, pellet-like forms are made of hardened bile or cholesterol. Pancreatic inflammation usually results from one of two gallstones happenings: 1) a gallstone that is passing through the common bile duct irritates the pancreas; 2) a gallstone becomes stuck in the biliary tract and thus blocks the exit of enzymes from the pancreas.

The following is a list of possible causes:

- alcoholism
- heredity/genetics
- certain medications
- high triglyceride levels in the blood (hypertriglyceridemia)
- high calcium levels in the blood (hypercalcemia), which may be caused by an overactive parathyroid gland (hyperparathyroidism)
- pancreatic cancer
- abdominal surgery
- cystic fibrosis
- infection
- injury to the abdomen
- obesity
- trauma

It's important to note that in some people with chronic pancreatitis, the cause cannot be identified. This is called *idiopathic* pancreatitis.

What is necrotizing pancreatitis?

When damage to the pancreas is severe, parts of your pancreas may not receive enough blood and oxygen to survive. This results in these areas dying off. If this dead tissue gets infected, it can cause serious issues. This affects the symptoms you may be experiencing and the type of treatment you will receive.

What causes necrotizing pancreatitis?

- high levels of blood fats (cholesterol)
- trauma to the pancreas
- pancreatic tumor
- high calcium levels in your blood
- autoimmune diseases
- damage to the pancreas from medicines
- hereditary conditions that harm the pancreas, e.g., cystic fibrosis

How is necrotizing pancreatitis diagnosed?

Diagnosing necrotizing pancreatitis involves a thorough evaluation by your doctor in order to understand your health history, symptoms, and any pre-existing conditions. You will be given an exam and also various tests to check your blood for enzymes, glucose, and other indicators. Any visual anomalies will be examined using an MRI, abdominal ultrasound, or CT scan. Physical samples of dead pancreatic tissue may also be taken with the use of a thin catheter inserted through your abdomen.

What is exocrine pancreatic insufficiency?

If the pancreas cannot produce enough enzymes, food cannot be digested properly. This medical condition is referred to as exocrine pancreatic insufficiency (EPI). When this is the case, your medical practitioner may prescribe creon. Creon serves as a replacement for the enzymes that your pancreas is no longer making, thus helping you to digest the fats, proteins, and carbohydrates (sugars) in food.

Chapter 3 - Takeaways

1. Your pancreas is an amazing organ. It plays a dual role, producing both digestive enzymes and hormones. Digestive enzymes do what you'd think, they aid in food digestion. The hormones, such as insulin, regulate blood sugar levels.
2. Understand the warning signs of this disease. By knowing the symptoms, such as severe abdominal pain, vomiting, and bloating, you can recognize potential health issues and seek timely medical attention.
3. If you think that you are having any of the symptoms of pancreatitis, seek immediate medical care. As I demonstrated with my personal story, this condition can be serious and potentially life-threatening. Delaying medical care may worsen the situation.

Chapter 4
HOW TO ACCESS VA AND NON-VA CARE

Before my first trip to the emergency room back in 2020, I typically only saw my primary care doctor once or twice a year for a checkup. The costs for these annual exams were covered by my civilian Blue Cross Blue Shield insurance. Yet after the medical procedures started piling up, and I could no longer work, this protection went away. But I wasn't worried. The VA would end up covering all my medical expenses. I hope the following information will help bring some clarity to your specific situation and how you can learn more about your VA benefits.

The first place to start is online. Visit the website for the U.S.Department of Veterans Affairs at www.va.gov. You can find a myriad of information. There are different tiers from 0 to 100%. First, you must be honorably discharged from one of the United States Armed Forces. Second, you must apply for VA health care and prescriptions. You are not automatically enrolled for these benefits. You must sign up.

The following couple of excerpts regarding health care come directly from the VA site:

What care and services does the Veterans Affairs health care cover?

Each Veteran's medical benefits package is unique. Yours will include care and services to help:

- treat illnesses, and injuries.
- prevent future health problems.
- improve your ability to function.
- enhance your quality of life.

All Veterans receive coverage for most care and services, but only some will qualify for added benefits such as dental care. The full list of your covered benefits depends on:

- your priority group.
- the advice of your VA primary care provider (your main doctor, nurse practitioner, or physician's assistant).
- the medical standards for treating any health conditions you may have.

If you are disabled, you can see what benefits you and your family might receive, from a 10% up to 100% rating for service-connected disability. Speak with Eligibility at your nearest VA facility, call 1(800)-MyVA-411, or go to:

https://www.va.gov/disability/compensation-rates/veteran-rates/

How is VA care different from non-VA care?

VA care is exclusively available to all Veterans who have served honorably in the United States military. When seeking help for non-emergency related services, you will need to locate your nearest VA health facility or VA-approved location. Your benefits do not cover non-VA care unless your condition is life-threatening or you meet certain eligibility criteria.

Think you might have pancreatitis? Use this prep list and bring it with you to your doctor visit.

1. Write down any symptoms that you might be experiencing.
2. What time and date did you experience them.
3. What is going on when these symptoms happen?
4. Any other pertinent details?
5. Call your primary care medical team to set an appointment with your VA doctor to get checked out.
6. Bring your list of symptoms with you so you remember clearly. The clearer you are, the more your doctor can help you figure things out.

Do you need help right away?

Urgent Care. If you are registered with the VA and have seen your primary care provider within the last twenty-four (24) months, you are eligible for VA's urgent care benefit.

You can visit an in-network urgent care clinic to treat minor injuries and illnesses that are not life-threatening. To verify your eligibility for VA urgent care, call your primary care team.

Emergency Care. During a medical emergency, you should immediately seek care at the nearest hospital, whether it is a VA medical center or not. Veterans do not need to check with VA before calling an ambulance or going to a community hospital emergency department. However, for the VA to coordinate and potentially pay for emergency care, you must notify them within seventy-two (72) hours of your clinic and/or hospital visit.

If you have an immediate medical concern in regards to pancreatitis, don't wait. Symptoms can include fever, nausea, vomiting, elevated heart rate, but especially sharp, stabbing abdominal pain. Seek immediate medical attention at your local emergency room, VA or non-VA medical clinic, or VA or non-VA hospital.

If you are admitted to a non-VA hospital emergency room, you can always request to be transported to a VA hospital. If not, let your VA Community Care program know within 24-72 hours, where you are, so that the VA can pay your hospital bills. Pursuant to Title I of the Maintaining Internal Systems and Strengthening Integrated Outside Networks Act of 2018, Veterans are eligible to receive health care at non-VA medical facilities, if they meet the eligibility criteria.

If the VA is unable to provide the care you need, the VA Office of Community Care can connect you through its Community Care Network (CCN) with non-VA community providers. This is based on your eligibility, your specific needs, and the availability of (or lack thereof) the specific VA care you require.

The Office of Community Care offers these services:

- consultation and review
- scheduling authorization
- community care visit
- scheduling additional appointments
- prescription reauthorization
- durable medical equipment pick-up
- receiving and paying your bill

If you are a Veteran who has served honorably in the United States military, then the bottom line is this, you are eligible for VA benefits. Please be proactive with your health.

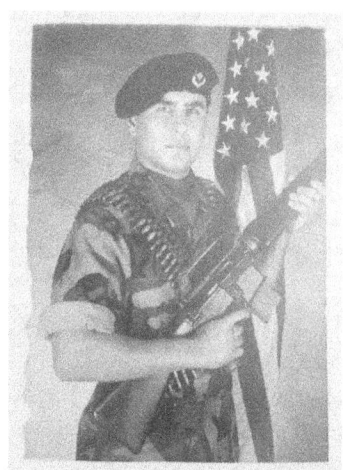

Chapter 4 - Takeaways:

1. VA care is available to all honorably discharged Veterans.
2. Long before you are ever faced with a potentially life-threatening situation, do your research. Be informed and up-to-date on what your VA benefits are.
3. For emergency care, Veterans should immediately seek treatment at the nearest hospital, whether it is a VA medical center or not. The VA should be notified within 72 hours of the visit to potentially coordinate and pay for emergency care.
4. If the VA is unable to provide the required care, you can access the VA Office of Community Care, which can connect you to non-VA community providers based on eligibility and specific needs.
5. Know where your nearest VA medical facilities are located. VA clinic, VA hospital, VA emergency room, and non-VA emergency room. Be sure to keep this information with your ID.

Chapter 5
HOW TO FOLLOW UP WITH YOUR PRIMARY CARE MEDICAL TEAM

Take ownership of your own health. As I've repeated throughout this book, please be proactive. Don't just leave it up to your doctors, nurses, and other staff to follow-up with you. Contact your local VA if you have questions, need more details, or you think something is wrong. Do not wait for the doctor to tell you what to do. If you are having symptoms, go get them checked out. Do not take no for an answer.

If you don't know who to talk to, ask who you should call to find out. You will be pointed in the right direction. Also ask if there are any forms you might need to complete and, if so, where you should submit them. Check online at www.va.gov for additional information.

The VA has many programs available to help all eligible Veterans. They do vary by state, so please check within your own to see what is available to you in your location.

Try to always make your scheduled appointment. Be at least fifteen minutes early. If you have to cancel, do so by text, e-mail, or phone call at least twenty-four hours before your appointment time, thus allowing another Veteran to fill your canceled spot.

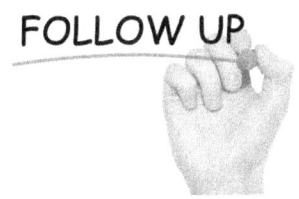

FOLLOW UP

Top ten tips to get the most from your follow-up visit with your primary healthcare provider:

1. Know the reason for your visit, and what you want to happen.
2. Before the appointment, make a list of questions and concerns you want to discuss. This ensures you cover all the important topics during your visit.
3. Bring someone with you to help ask questions and to remember what your provider tells you. Alternatively, during the appointment, take notes or ask if you can record the conversation. This way you can review the information later and follow your provider's recommendations more effectively.
4. Bring with you a list of symptoms you're experiencing. Describe these symptoms in detail. Include information about the duration,

frequency, and any triggers or patterns you've
noticed.

5. At the visit, write down the name of any new
   diagnosis, any new medicines, treatments, or
   tests. Also write down any new instructions
   your provider gives you.

6. Be sure you know why a new medicine or
   treatment is prescribed and how it might help
   you. Also know what the side effects are. Ask
   what to expect if you do not take the medicine,
   if you don't do the test, or if you choose not to
   have the procedure.

7. Ask if your condition can be treated in other
   ways.

8. Be sure you know why a test or procedure is
   recommended and what the results could mean.

9. Before leaving, make sure you understand the
   next steps in your treatment plan. Ask about
   follow-up appointments, referrals, or any
   further tests or procedures. Write down the
   time, date, and the purpose for that visit before
   you leave.

10. Get contact information for your primary care
    provider team (doctor, nurse, and staff) in case
    you should have any questions, comments, or
    concerns later on.

Chapter 5 - Takeaways

1. Be proactive with your own health and recovery.
2. Do not be afraid (or too proud) to ask for help.
3. Do utilize every service available to you.
4. Follow through with all of the medical advice given from your medical team of doctors, nurses, and staff.

Chapter 6
HOW HAS MY LIFE CHANGED?

My life after having severe, life-threatening CNP, and now living with type-2 diabetes, has not been all sunshine and roses. Yet, researching, writing, and publishing my story has truly helped me with my mental therapy. Many areas of my life are getting back to some normalcy. I still have difficulty with certain tasks, but I just focus on my desire to thrive.

Now that I am considered 100% disabled by the VA, I feel blessed that I no longer have to chase a W-2 job, especially since I physically would not be able to sustain a 40-hour work week anymore. My mindset has now shifted to working for myself and helping others by sharing my story and experience. A law school, two universities, and a tribal college have all reached out, asking me to teach courses to their students. I am now teaching part-time, working virtually from my home.

The recovery continues. Recently, Juanita and Justice were able to visit family in New Mexico for the weekend and leave me home alone. This is a big deal and wasn't something that was possible even six months ago.

First, and foremost, I am focusing on improving my

health even more. It's been a slow but steady climb. I want to be present and the healthiest that I can for the next fifty years. I want to walk Justice down the aisle as she gets married. I want to be present in the lives of my grandchildren and great-grandchildren.

My diet has changed drastically, but for the better. I am now eating healthier and more smartly. No longer do I consume greasy junk foods, candy, and soda pop. I drink a lot of good clean water. With the help of a dietitian RN, I've learned that I need to eat at least 20 grams of protein per meal and less than 20 grams of carbs. Along with this, I have two snacks of 10 grams of protein every day.

I have been assigned by the VA a diabetes RN who helps me check my blood sugar. I do this at least four times a day with a Freestyle Libre 14-day glucose sensor.

My mission now is to share with you, other Veterans, my path to recovery to help you to do the same. At present, my health has stabilized.

I now consider myself a "professional patient," but it was not always this way. Prior to December 12, 2020–when I woke up to that spinning room–my mindset was completely different. I never enjoyed going to any clinic or hospital. But now, I accept that challenge. I want my health to continue to improve. Not only for myself but especially for my children, my grandchildren, and future great-grandchildren. So therefore, I am continually, and closely being watched by the Yukon VA clinic's primary care medical team, along with the OKC VAMC Medical Center specialty clinics.

We are not guaranteed one minute into the future. We cannot get back one second from the past. All we have is this moment. The here. The now. Every single day is a precious gift from God. Be present. It's up to you to take the initiative to help yourself. You are worth it. If you are here in this world, then you still have time left. It's worth the effort to make your life better. If you raise the quality of your own life, it will help to improve the lives of everyone around you as well.

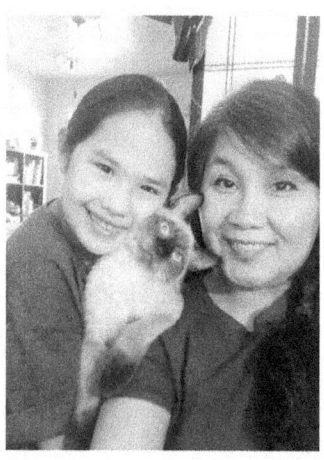

Despite the challenges and setbacks I faced during this healing journey, I want to leave you with a message of hope. With dedication, perseverance, and the support of medical professionals, support groups, your friends, and loved ones, it is possible to reclaim one's life and regain a sense of normalcy. Healing may take time, and there might be moments of doubt and difficulty, but it is possible to overcome health obstacles and find a way to live a fulfilling life again. The path to recovery may be challenging, but the potential for a brighter future is attainable for you too.

Chapter 6 - Takeaways:

1. Embrace resilience and hope. Your life after facing pancreatitis may not be all easy, but remember that you can find the strength to overcome these challenges.
2. Value your future. Your determination to improve your health is driven by your own *why*. Keep it ever in mind to motivate you to seek medical care and maintain stability.
3. Seize the present moment. Remember, every single day is a precious gift. Dedicate yourself to healing and recovery, and with the help of medical professionals, support groups, friends, and loved ones, you will regain a new sense of normalcy.
4. Envision a brighter future.

ONE LAST MESSAGE

Congratulations! I am so proud of you for making the great decision to better yourself. I truly admire and respect you for wanting to improve your health, your personal growth, and your way of life.

Remember, learning in any particular subject matter is an ongoing process. You should always try to expand your knowledge everyday. My hope is that you become more inspired to live your life to the fullest, no matter where you are along your healing journey. You can do it!

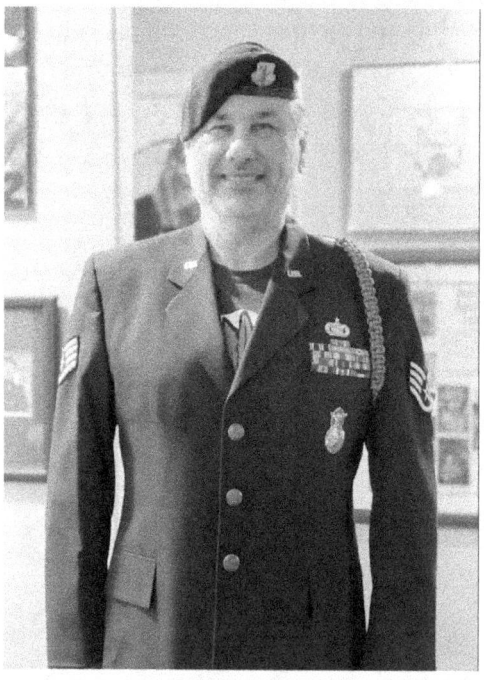

RESOURCES

Books and References:

Coenegrachts, Kenneth; Hans, Rigauts; De Wilde, Vincent; Denolin, Vincent. Diagnosis and Imaging of Chronic Pancreatitis. Nova Science Publishers, Inc, 2011.

Dagradi, A.; Scuro, L.A.; Marzoli, G.P.; Cavallini, G.; Pederzoli, P., and Banterte, C. Topics in Acute and Chronic Pancreatitis. Springer, 1981.

Harlow, Sylvia. Acute and Chronic Pancreatitis. Foster Academics, 2019.

Li, Zhao-Shen; Liao, Zhuan; Chen, Jian-Min; Ferec, Claude. Chronic Pancreatitis: From Basic Research to Clinical Treatment. Springer, 2017.

Poltrona, Tony. The Pancreatitis Handbook: An Easy-To-Read Guide. CreateSpace Independent Publishing Platform, 2012.

Self-Care Skills for the Person with Diabetes: VA/DoD Clinical Practice Guideline for Management of Diabetes Mellitus, Version 4. 2010.

VA Healthy Teaching Kitchen. Nutrition and Food Services, 2022.

VA MOVE Weight Management Program for Veterans Workbook and Curriculum, National Institute of Diabetes and Digestive and Kidney Disease, 2019.

Rush, Sharon. Pancreatitis Diet Cookbook: The 5-Step Beginner's Guide to Help You Manage & Control Pancreatitis with 400 Quick & Easy Recipes, Workouts, and a 28-Day Step-By-Step Diet Plan for a Healthy Living. 2022.

**These are just a few of the many books available on pancreatitis, healthy diets, and related issues. Check your local bookstore or online for more titles.

Articles

Kovalska, Dronov, Zemskov, Deneka, Zemskova. "Patterns of Pathomorphological Changes in Acute Necrotizing Pancreatitis." International Journal of Inflammation. Kylanpaa, 2012.

VA Health Care System Veteran Newsletter.

Podcasts:

You can find many good podcasts online that address pancreatitis and related issues, including healthy diets and other helpful information. Simply do a keyword search on your favorite podcast platform.

Videos:

What Can I Expect Following the Diagnosis of Chronic Pancreatitis?

https://youtu.be/r-YvXCnz4uo

Pancreatitis: Causes, Symptoms, Treatments, and More
https://youtu.be/pL-NilzVoSU

What Does the Pancreas Do?
https://youtu.be/8dgoeYPoE-o

Pancreatitis: Acute and Chronic Pancreatitis Nursing Lecture Symptoms, Treatment, Pathophysiology
https://youtu.be/deT4TeBsmbc

Free: Brand New Medical Supplies & Equipment
https://youtu.be/gGXFIDsTzfI

Websites

www.va.gov

www.move.va.gov

www.nutrition.va.gov

ACKNOWLEDGMENTS

First, and foremost, Chi-Migwetch/Kitahtahmiin Ki-Si-Mahn-To (I am really thankful very much God, the Creator of us all). I am so grateful to be alive, and fortunate for all the blessings in my life. Looking back over my life, I have been truly blessed.

Second, I want to acknowledge Chi-Migwetch Kitah-tahmiin (thank you in Anishanaabe and NeIyahw) Nizhoni (beautiful in Dine) NiChiMos, my wifey, Juanita Benally Morsette for her faith, hope, and love. In my mind, she is my angel. She rushed me to the emergency room on two-separate occasions, and saved my life within an hour of dying both times respectively. She is my honorary registered nurse practitioner that nursed me back to health each, and every day.

Third, I want to acknowledge that it takes a large medical team to help me get well. Therefore, I want to acknowledge all of the Doctors, Nurses, and Staff from Rocky Boy Tribal Health, White Earth Health Center, Meskwaki Nation Health Clinic, Grand Forks VA Clinic, Fargo VA Health Care, Marshalltown VA Clinic, Des Moines VA Medical Center, El Reno Indian Health Services, Clinton Indian Health Service, Yukon Emergency Room, Integris Canadian Valley Hospital, Oklahoma City VA Emergency Room and Health Care and Hospital, Yukon VA Clinic, and Oklahoma University Medical

Center Emergency Room, Health Care, and Hospital; and special recognition to Guy Hicks Jr. who was a roommate to me at the OKC VA Hospital, (RIP).

SPECIAL FREE BONUS GIFTS FOR YOU

To help you to achieve more success, there are

FREE BONUS RESOURCES for you at:

www.HighEagleLLC.com/free-gifts

ABOUT JOSEPH

Joseph Henry Morsette, MSCJA, JD, LL.M., Is-Pi-Mik-Ki-Ew (High Eagle) is a #1 Bestselling author, course-creator, coach, and an inspirational speaker. He is an enrolled member (non-allottee) of Ogimah Ahsniiwin Chief Rocky Boy's Band of Anishinaabe (in English aka Ojibwe or Chippewa) and such other homeless Indians in the State of Montana as the Secretary of the Interior may see fit to locate thereon [see the United States Department of the Interior, Bureau of Indian Affairs, Federal Registry, Chippewa Cree Indians of the Rocky Boy's Reservation, Montana (previously listed as Chippewa Cree Indians of the Rocky Boy's Reservation, Montana)]; descendant of the Cherokee Nation; and Canadian French. Joseph has delivered hundreds of presentations for tribal, and state programs, tribal citizens, high schools, colleges, universities, and law schools throughout the United States, and in Canada. Joseph can speak for groups ranging from one to thousands [in person, and on social media, such as zoom].

www.HighEagleLLC.com

Mr. Morsette has come full-circle, from being the student and graduating from his alma mater, Stone Child College; to continuing to teach, at present online courses, some that he developed from scratch, to researching, and writing his own books. His book series can be used at the other thirty-three tribal colleges and/or universities; or really any college and/or university that instructs their students on federal Indian law, tribal law and government, and taking a closer look at the tribal government and laws that impact the Rocky Boy's Indian Reservation. He is the first SCC alumnus to graduate with a Juris Doctorate (JD) (2009); and a Master of Laws (LL.M.) (2010). He was honored for his JD at Stone Child College's 25TH Anniversary (2009).

He has formerly taught NAS 253: History of Tribal Government of the Rocky Boy's Indian Reservation (required course); NAS 255: Indian Law (required course); Introduction to Tribal Legal Studies NAS 180 his proposed LS-100 course for SCC; Tribal Courts and Tribal Law NAS 180-02 his proposed LS-120 course for SCC; Criminal Law and Jurisdiction in Indian Country NAS 180-01 his proposed LS 210 course for SCC; Tribal Criminal Law and Procedure NAS 280 his proposed LS 130 course for SCC. He is currently an Adjunct Professor at Cameron University having taught Criminal Psychology. He has formerly taught tribal government (required course), civil jurisdiction in Indian country (elective course) at the University of Tulsa Law School in the online Master of Jurisprudence in Indian Law program; and formerly co-taught federal Indian law with Dean Kathryn Rand at the University of North Dakota School of Law.

Mr. Morsette set out on the educational path in criminal justice, in law, and academia to be best equipped, and prepared for a future career in education and training within his Native community in the field of tribal legal studies, and criminal justice studies.

Mr. Morsette is a Fellowship Award Recipient from the James E. Rogers College of Law University of Arizona, and was conferred a Master of Laws (LL.M.) degree in Indigenous Peoples Law & Policy; conferred a Juris Doctorate (JD) degree from the University of North Dakota School of Law; conferred with distinction a Master of Science in Criminal Justice Administration from the University of Great Falls; conferred a Bachelor of Sciences in Criminal Justice, Law Enforcement Concentration from the University of Great Falls; and conferred with distinction Associate of Arts, in Liberal Arts from Stone Child College.

Mr. Morsette's prior legal and criminal justice employment include: A Legal Consultant to the Executive Branch of the Cheyenne and Arapaho Tribes; the sole, in-house Legal Consultant to the Sixth-Ninth Legislature, Legislative Branch of the Cheyenne and Arapaho Tribes; Assistant Attorney General to the Sac and Fox Tribe of the Mississippi in Iowa (Meskwaki Nation) Tribal Council; Assistant Tribal prosecutor at Meskwaki Nation; Child Support Tribal Attorney for the Meskwaki Nation; Tribal Chief Judge and Chief Executive Officer (CEO) at Spirit Lake Nation; Tribal Associate Appellate Justice at White Earth Nation; Director of Recruitment and Retention of the Native Americans Into Law (NAIL) Program & the Faculty Fellow, Northern Plains Indian Law Center (NPILC) at the University of North Dakota School of Law; Tribal Associate Judge, and acting Chief Judge at Chippewa-Cree Tribe; Tribal Public Defender at Pascua Yaqui Tribe; Police Officer, Department of the Interior, Bureau of Indian Affairs, Law Enforcement Services; United States Air Force combat veteran of foreign wars (AFSC: 3PO71 Security Police); and United States Army (MOS: 19E trained on the M-48, M-60, and M1-Abraham Tanks).

Mr. Morsette is the Founder, and Owner of "High Eagle Legal Services," see the CCT Tribal Employment

Rights Ordinance of (2009), and now "High Eagle Coaching and Consulting Services, LLC" see the State of Oklahoma (2022): Training tribal court personnel, lay advocates, police officers, public officials, staff, and community members; contractual criminal defense; Judge pro tempore; and Adjunct Professor of tribal government, federal Indian law, tribal law and government, and criminal justice in Colleges and Universities online and on campus internationally. Mr. Morsette is the Founder of www.HighEagle LLC.com

Mr. Morsette teaches in the area of federal Indian law; tribal law; tribal government; tribal criminal law and procedure; criminal law and the courts; introduction to tribal legal studies, criminal jurisdiction in Indian country; civil jurisdiction in Indian country; tribal policing; introduction to law enforcement; police theory and practices; patrol operations and procedures; introduction to criminal justice system; field experience in law enforcement; community policing; criminal investigation; corrections and the Bureau of Indian Affairs law enforcement services; Indian Civil Rights Act of 1968 and its amendments; family law in Indian country; criminal evidence and procedure; psychology of criminal behavior; and police management. He is currently in the process of writing a tribal book series for tribal colleges and universities; starting with Stone Child College on the Rocky Boy's Indian Reservation.

www.HighEagleLLC.com

Other books by Joseph Morsette
INDIAN LAWS
BEST-KEPT SECRETS REVEALED

Audiobook more you style?
Listen as I narrate my book!

To order go to:
www.HighEagleLLC.com

Thank you for your order. Please contact customer support at www.HighEagleLLC.com if you have any questions, comments, and/or concerns about your order.

What is your shortcut to success, next steps?
If you would like to schedule summer courses; fall courses; spring courses; for a keynote and/or motivational speaking engagements; online courses; one, two, and/or three-day seminars, and/or webinars; workshop group training; working with you in a one-on-one coaching program; book signing tours; consulting training; know your rights training; codification training; reviewing and revising tribal constitutional training; reviewing and revising laws, ordinances, acts, and resolutions training; tribal court lay advocate training; Bridge Builder To Success Program and Courses – Certificate of Attendance, Certificate of Achievement, Certificate of Training, and/or Certificate of Completion Program; Train the Trainer; in-person, and/or zoom meetings: Mr. Morsette can be reached at www.HighEagle LLC.com

Special <u>FREE</u> Bonus Gifts for You
To help you to achieve more success, there are
FREE BONUS RESOURCES for you at:
www.HighEagleLLC.com/free-gifts

APPENDIX 1 - VA RESOURCES

The VA resources available to Veterans vary from state to state. Depending on where you live, you may have a slew of programs and treatments to choose from. Here in Oklahoma, this is an example of the VA health care services, departments, and facilities I tapped in to:

Oklahoma City VA Medical Center

- emergency room
- general surgery
- emergency intensive care unit
- intensive care unit
- overflow trailers
- gastroenterology
- physical therapy nurse
- occupational therapy nurse
- eye clinic
- monthly phone conferences regarding my blood pressure
- CPAP, which is automatically sent and reviewed by the VA at home video connect group for arthritis seated exercise recreational therapy, VA MOVE program, cooking program, and Tai Chi program

- cardiology
- radiology
- orthology
- orthotics and prosthetics
- urology
- podiatry
- My HealtheVet online service
- dental clinic

University of Oklahoma Medical Center

- specialty surgery
- emergency intensive care unit
- intensive care unit

Yukon VA clinic

- primary care
- physical therapy nurse
- occupational therapy nurse
- dietitian nurse
- diabetes nurse
- eye clinic
- cardiology
- audiology
- orthopedics

VA Community Care program

- orthotics and prosthetics
- surgery on my left shoulder

- physical therapy on my pelvic area
- physical therapy on my left shoulder
- bariatric surgery
- Home Health Care nurses and physical therapy nurses

APPENDIX 2 - ADDITIONAL PHOTOS

Before

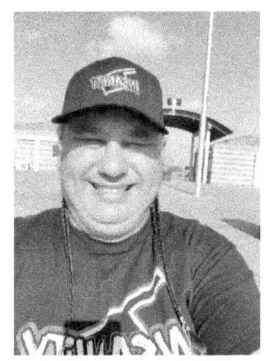

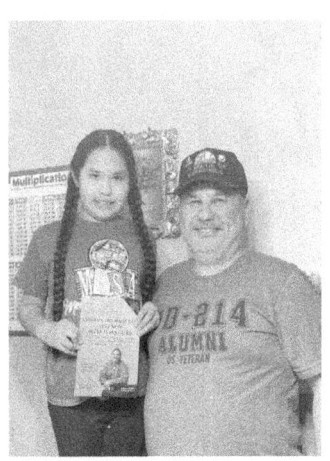

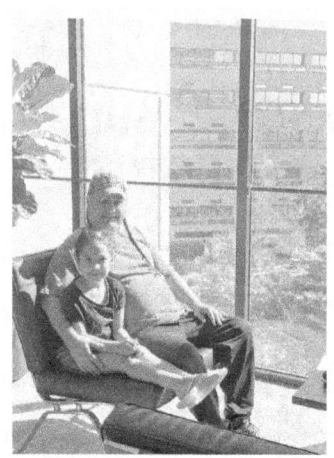

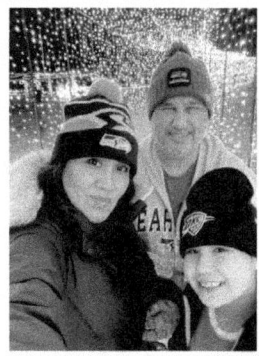

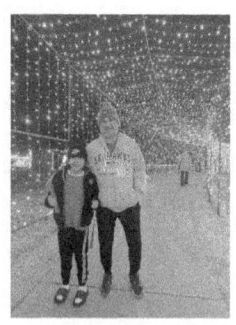

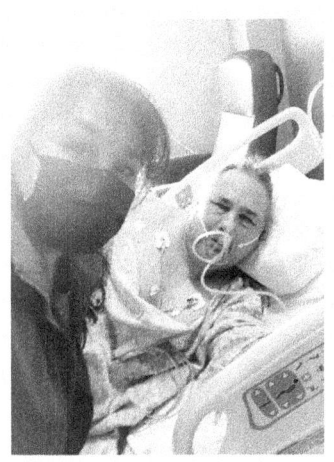

December 12, 2020

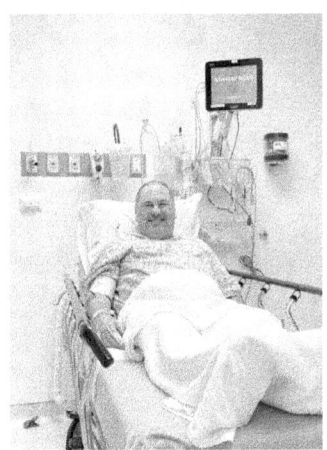

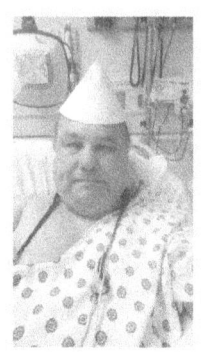

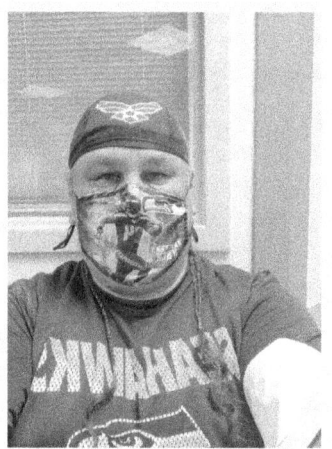

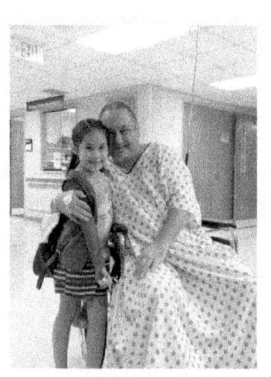

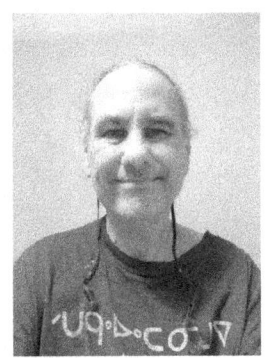

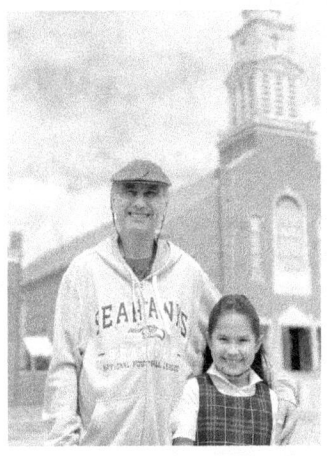

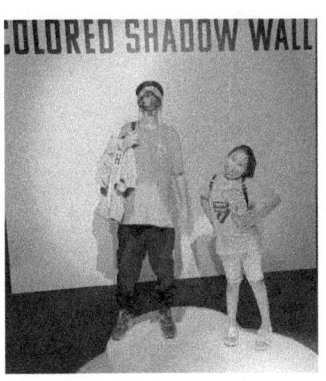

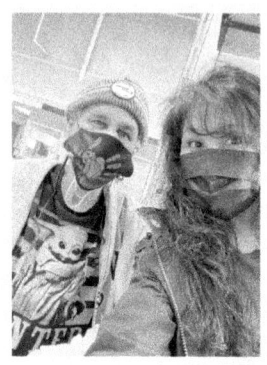

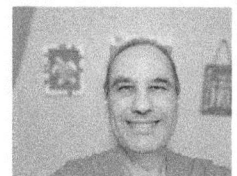

Losing my hair was especially hard on me.

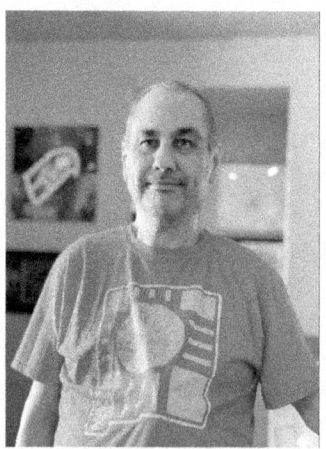

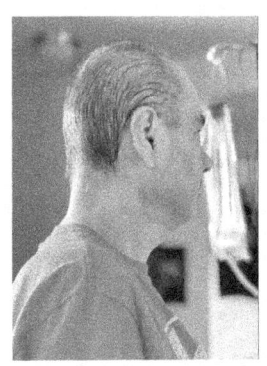

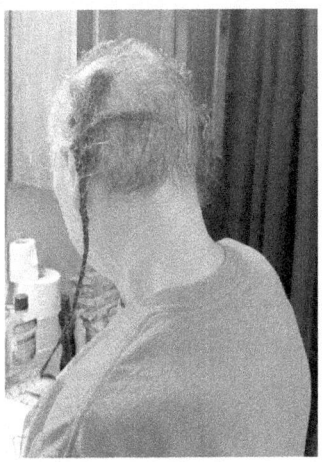

Last braid to go.

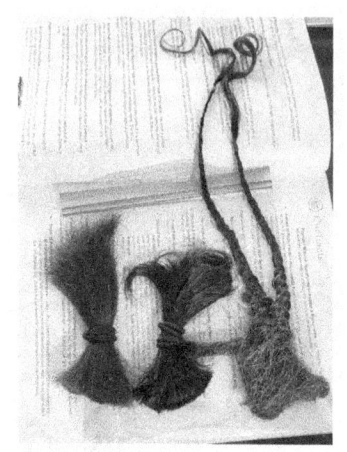

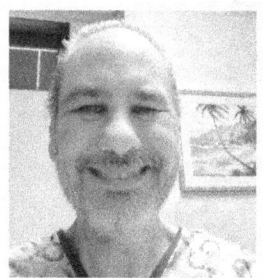

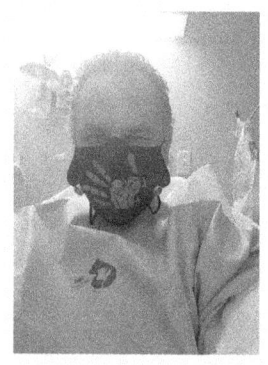

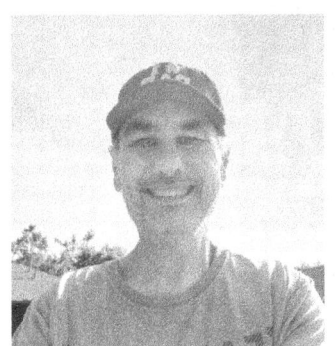

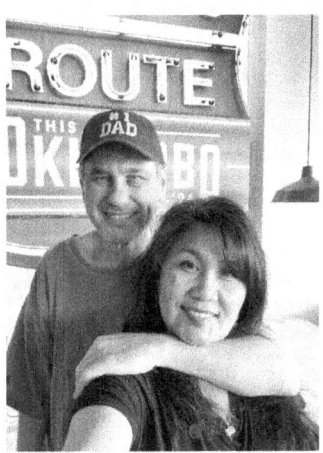

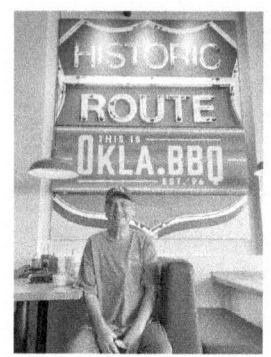

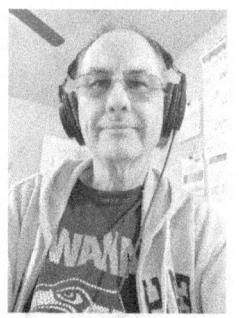

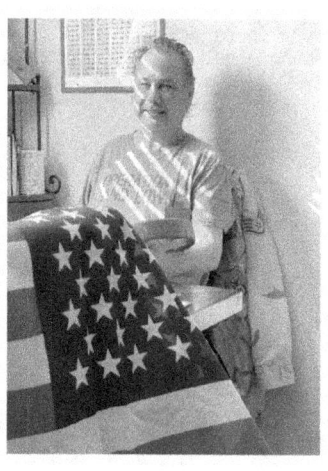

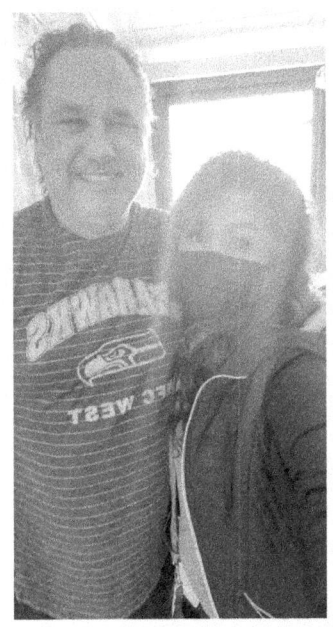

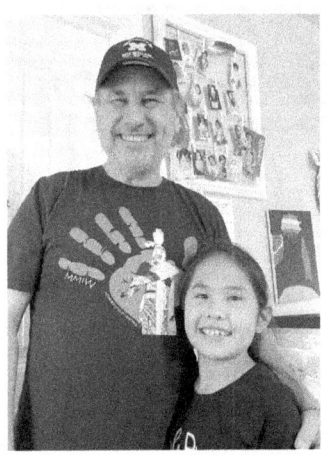

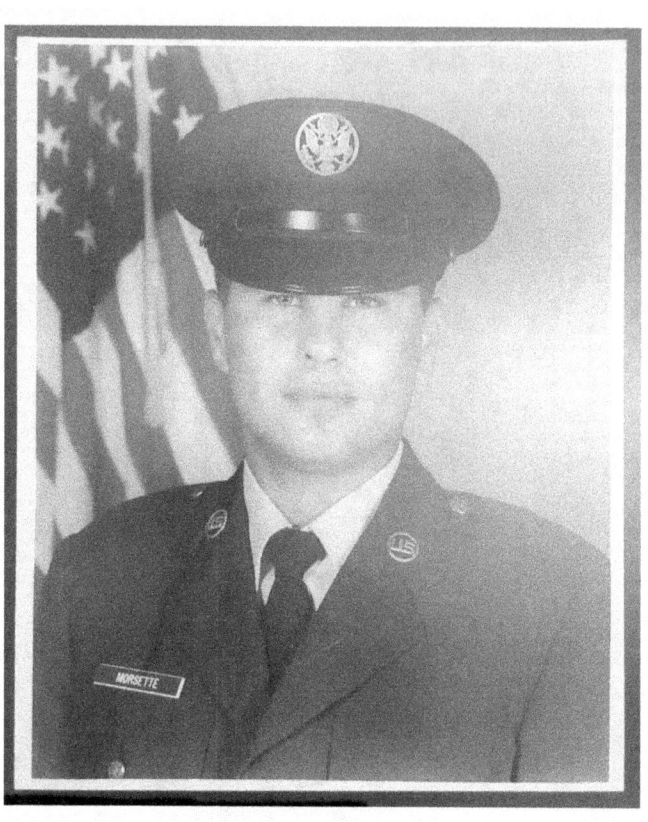